The 1918 Spanish Flu

The Tragic History of the Massive Influenza Outbreak

James Parker

licensed professional before attempting any techniques outlined in this book.

By reading this document, the reader agrees that under no circumstances is the author responsible for any losses, direct or indirect, which are incurred as a result of the use of information contained within this document, including, but not limited to, — errors, omissions, or inaccuracies.

TABLE OF CONTENTS

Introduction 1
Why is it so hard to pin down the death toll? 4
Disease at the Turn of the 19th Century............................5
Influenza is always potentially fatal.................................8
Terms to Know 9

What is Influenza?...11
Meet the Influenza Virus 13
Leading Up to the Spanish Flu: The Russian Flu Epidemic
of 1889...14

The Spanish Flu...17
Where did it come from? 17
China 18
The United Kingdom, care of France 19
The United States, and the Men of Haskell County, Kansas
....20
The Infection of Europe: Spring 1918 23

**The Second Wave and the Deadliest Year of the
Century**...27
The Mutation 27
The Second Wave in the United States 29
Carry a Potato in Your Pocket...30
Medical Mysteries During the Spanish Flu......................32
The Unexpected Affliction of Young Adults and the
Cytokine Storm..32
The Theory of Aspirin Poisoning 34
Countermeasures...35
Philadelphia: The Pandemic's Most Devastating Example
....38

The Long Ending **44**
Armistice and the Third Wave 44
Medical Advances Made During the Spanish Flu Pandemic
....46
A Silver Lining: Women's Increased Status in the Fallout of
Flu and War 48

Stories from the Spanish Flu **50**

The "Forgotten Pandemic"? **56**

Biological Warfare: Outing the Spanish Flu **58**
The Research that Followed 58
Finding the Real Spanish Flu Virus 61
Why is the genetic sequencing important? 64
Creating a Lethal Virus 65
The Live Virus: Available for Interrogation 67
What was learned from the reconstructed virus? 68

One Hundred Years Since Then **70**
How Safe Are We From an Influenza Pandemic? 72

Conclusion: Centennial **76**

Resources **77**
Films 77
Books/Articles 77
Websites 79

Introduction

The Spanish Lady. Three-Day Fever. Sandfly Fever. Blitz Katarrh. The Blue Death. The Spanish Flu. These were some of the names given to a pandemic that, for almost two years, gripped the world. This is the bizarre horror story of a disease, deadly and fast-moving, that was often ignored in favor of feeding a war machine engaged in worldwide conflict. Once the pandemic had lifted, memory of it was pushed out of the public mind, as if the whole thing were simply too baffling and chaotic to recall.

From January 1918 until December 1920, as people around the world focused on the final stages of World War I, a strain of influenza virus (Influenza A virus subtype H1N1) crawled across the globe, carried on the backs of soldiers, transported by ships across every ocean, bolstered by increases in civilian travel and a general failure of sanitation and public health safety. It was the deadliest flu pandemic in history. Due to a strange twist of fate concerning wartime censorship, the illness was dubbed the "Spanish Flu" although it gathered other frightening nicknames as time passed. Roughly one-third of the world's population was infected, a fraction that, at the time, meant about 500 million people contracted the illness.

The Spanish Flu moved fast, over two years and in three "waves."

The First Wave (Spring 1918) was a severe and highly contagious influenza spread into the trenches of war in Europe.

There, at some point during the summer of 1918, the virus mutated into something so strange and deadly that it could hardly be identified, much less contained, in the **Second Wave (Fall 1918).** This mutation is responsible for the majority of the Spanish Flu fatalities as well as much of the fallout of financial and social devastation.

Then in late 1918, and again for unknown reasons, the virus mutated once more, into a less deadly form. This ***Third Wave (Winter 1918 until approximately December 1920)*** *was able to cause widespread illness and continued fatalities, but not nearly at the terrifying and uncontrolled levels of the Second Wave.*

That the flu was devastating is not in doubt, but the exact number of deaths has never been decisively calculated. Estimates of the numbers of global deaths range from 17 million to as high as 100 million. In general, the approximation of 50 million deaths is considered the "best guess." The exact number of deaths is impossible to know due to poor record keeping, particularly during the most deadly months of the Second Wave.

Now over a hundred years after the Spanish Flu pandemic, perhaps the most disturbing fact is that the virus (H1N1) still exists, having emerged once more in 2009's swine flu epidemic, causing the deaths of more than 12,000 Americans. As it is an existing biohazard, all aspects of the Spanish Flu of 1918 are considered valuable areas of study, from the genetic mapping of the virus to discover its traits and develop vaccines, to the methods employed to curb the spread -- or those that should have been employed but were not.

To this day, the CDC considers Influenza A virus subtype H1N1 a biosecurity and biosafety threat.

In 1918, the world seemed to be a personal invitation to a deadly virus, a perfect combination of population movement and chaos that resulted in pandemic. As we proceed, we'll discuss the Spanish Flu and its far-reaching effects through the world and time.

Why is it so hard to pin down the death toll?

No research seems to agree on the number of worldwide deaths actually caused by the Spanish Flu. An approximation of at least 50 million deaths worldwide seems to be the closest experts can come to agreement, usually with the caveat that "it was probably a lot more than that."

The broad guesswork of the Spanish Flu death toll (ranging from 17 million deaths to 100 million) can be blamed on a variety of reasons, not the least of which is that record-keeping was imperfect at best, and vastly different depending on the part of the world taking the measurements.

Studies that attempt to pinpoint a number are criticized for incomplete records and flawed methodology. In a listing of countries that were actually keeping track, the estimates normally quantify their findings with "At least 'x' number of people died from the flu" meaning that a total count would be impossible to ascertain.

The United States did fairly well in the keeping of records, or at least in making them subsequently available, so its totals are more precise. But no one seems able to really pin down the fatalities of the Second Wave. During the hellish weeks of September through November 1918, health care workers could begin a workday healthy and be deathly ill by that evening, as the fast-moving virus could kill in as little as twelve hours. It was all that even professional medical staff could do to care for themselves and the sick, but in many cases the ranks of caregivers had to be filled by students and volunteers. Record-keeping was a secondary consideration at best.

It is also unknown exactly how long the virus was active as it was initially often misdiagnosed, due to its unusual symptoms (including hemorrhaging of mucus membranes, a symptom normally seen in cholera or typhoid rather than the flu). In many cases, early outbreaks were not identified as influenza at all, due to the bizarre and unprecedented symptoms presenting in the Second Wave's mutation. And, while the flu itself could kill victims through hemorrhaging or lung edema, a significant number of deaths were caused secondarily by pneumonia or a bacterial superinfection. Therefore, it is currently impossible to know how many of those deaths were correctly linked to the Spanish Flu.

Disease at the Turn of the 19th Century

Contagious disease happens when people live together. Some 10,000 years ago, humanity moved to an agrarian lifestyle that created community life, and contagious disease has been a part of our existence since that time. Our early ancestors lived, and died, not just with influenza, but with smallpox, tuberculosis, leprosy, and malaria. With every move forward in civilization (trading, roads, and cities) came new opportunities for disease to spread. In the 14th Century, the Black Death killed a significant chunk of the world's population - estimates range from 75 to 200 million people succumbing before the pandemic ended.

Too much contagious disease leads to social change. Looking at the turn of the 19th Century and the decades immediately following, we find a world that was fairly accustomed to outbreaks of contagious diseases. The Industrial Revolution had caused a dreadful downward shift in public health, as cities grew exponentially and people were crowded into smaller and smaller spaces. Finally, in the mid-19th century, the outcry of health care officials and workers could no longer be ignored as life expectancies plummeted and infant mortality skyrocketed. By sheer necessity, public health had been slowly but steadily improving since around 1850, with cities taking more care to ensure that clean water and sanitation were available, while also encouraging healthy eating. Germs had been discovered to exist, leading to new techniques in cleanliness as well as methods for staving off the spread of disease.

Medical technology had not yet discovered penicillin or antibiotics, and the existence of viruses was unknown. Diseases were treated by trying to alleviate the symptoms; little else could be done.

In the 19th and early 20th century, epidemics from the following diseases were rather common:

1. **Diphtheria.** Diphtheria is a bacterial infection that, through swelling of the neck and throat, and coating of the mucus membranes, can cause severe difficulty swallowing and/or breathing. In the 1920s, diphtheria yearly caused thirteen to fifteen thousand deaths; a majority of its victims were children.

2. **Cholera.** Cholera is a bacterial infection of the lower intestine characterized mostly by severe diarrhea, that results in dehydration so severe that it can be deadly. Many of us now are familiar with cholera as a way to die while playing the *The Oregon Trail*, but it is still an active killer in some parts of the world where clean water is an unknown luxury.

3. **Yellow Fever**. Yellow fever is a viral disease with almost exactly the same symptoms as flu, but that is contracted from mosquito bites

4. **Typhoid Fever**. Typhoid fever is a bacterial infection that has similar symptoms to flu (except these symptoms seldom include diarrhea). Like cholera, typhoid fever can be caused by unsanitary drinking water and conditions.

An interesting fact about these four diseases is that when it seized the United States, the Spanish Flu was, at some point and in various places, mistaken for all four of them.

Influenza is always potentially fatal.

Looking at Center for Disease Control (CDC) charts of the leading causes of death in the United States from 1900 through 1917, one can see that pneumonia and influenza (always listed together) are invariably in the top three causes, along with tuberculosis and, usually, diseases of the heart. These three conditions trade places over the years but seldom allow any other causes to break into the medal-winning spots -- when another cause of death does manage to sneak in, it replaces heart disease, leaving influenza/pneumonia and tuberculosis still somewhere in their top three spots.

So there you have it: the flu, and the secondary pneumonia that came with it, was a leading cause of death for the two decades that preceded the 1918 pandemic. While it may no longer be a leading cause of death, each year, even now, people die from flu complications. Death from influenza has occurred for centuries, and it is certainly not a thing of the past.

The difference between yearly influenza and the pandemic of 1918, or any influenza pandemic, is a matter of morbidity and mortality. To begin understanding what it takes to turn a yearly cycle into a worldwide catastrophe, let's look at the seasonal flu, and what science now knows about influenza's workings.

Terms to Know

In discussing influenza and its spread, here are a few helpful terms to understand:

Antigenic Shift: An antigenic shift is a major change in a virus's genes that results in a "new" kind of influenza. An antigenic shift is dangerous because it decreases immunity. Here is how this happens: If you suffer but then recover from the flu, you develop antibodies against the virus that will prevent you from becoming ill again from *that* virus. But if that virus undergoes an antigenic shift, its genetic structure can change so much that your antibodies cannot recognize or fight it. The most devastating antigenic shift occurs when an animal-origin virus gains the ability to transmit to humans (think of bird flu, swine flu): humans have had no opportunity to develop immunity. Antigenic shifts can result in pandemics.

H__N__ Viruses: This is a way of referring to and numbering mutations of Influenza Virus A. The "H" stands for hemagglutinin protein and the "N" represents neuraminidase protein. Thus, we get Influenza viruses tagged as H1N1 (which was the virus type of the Spanish Flu), H3N2, H7N9, and so on.

Epidemic versus Pandemic: An epidemic is a disease outbreak that affects a large number of people in a particular group. This group could be a certain population or community of people, or could live in a particular geographical region. A pandemic is an epidemic that has spread across populations, communities, or throughout the world, crossing borders and continents.

Morbidity versus Mortality: Morbidity refers to the number of occurrences of the disease - *not* to fatalities from the disease. A flu with a high morbidity has many more infected victims. The *mortality* rate refers to the number of deaths resulting from a disease. Morbidity does not necessarily lead to mortality; it is simply the presence of ill health.

Transmissibility: This term concerns how easily a disease can be passed from one organism to another. An influenza virus with greater transmissibility results in a higher morbidity. As an example, currently the avian flu, or bird flu, is a dangerous influenza virus with a high rate of mortality. It is, however, not easily transmissible from human to human; mostly it affects humans who interact frequently with birds (poultry farmers, etc.). Its lack of transmissibility has kept it from becoming a pandemic.

What is Influenza?

Or, "Wait, don't we get this every year?"

First things first. Influenza (or "the flu," as we usually say) is a virus that attacks the respiratory system. It's usually quite easy to spread this virus from organism to organism, person to person. A virus is a living organism and as such, its purpose is to thrive and reproduce in the comfortable environment of your body, and then spread its offspring to as many other comfortable bodies as it can. Most of us are fully aware that transmission of an influenza virus can be accomplished through both physical contact and airborne particles. Shared surfaces (doorknobs, elevator buttons, or any number of surfaces in public areas) are prime grounds for transmission. When an infected person sneezes, coughs, or speaks, infected particles disperse into the surrounding air, which are breathed in by others.

This knowledge seems obvious and constant in our society. Each year in the fall, when school is back in session, a flu season begins; the flu season in the United States is, in general, from late fall to springtime. Vaccinations are available, with varying effectiveness. But some people each year will get the flu regardless of precautions. At times, seasonal influenza can result in complications, such as secondary pneumonia, and can be fatal, particularly to those with compromised immune systems, asthma, heart disease, and diabetes, and the two least-robust age groups: the very young and the very old. The Centers for Disease Control calculates that during an ordinary year, roughly 200,000 Americans will be hospitalized for complications from the flu, which includes conditions such as ear and sinus infections, bronchitis and pneumonia. The number of flu-related deaths varies from year to year, and over the last thirty years, the United States annually has suffered a death toll of 3,000 to 49,000 flu-related deaths.

The severity of any given flu season in the *current* era depends on three factors:

1. Which strain of flu is being spread?
2. How closely the available flu vaccine matches the year's strain of the flu?
3. How many people actually received the vaccination?

Obviously in 1918, the second two factors could not apply -- they did not have vaccinations to give out. But the passage of time only protects us so much, and only from seasonal flu severity and transmissibility. Living one hundred years later, with seasonal vaccines available, does not protect us from the same possible pandemic outcome, because pandemics arise when a *new* type of flu virus emerges for which there is little or no human immunity and no available vaccine.

So, let us now look at the reasons why a pandemic occurs, from the viral viewpoint:

Meet the Influenza Virus

Human influenza viruses come in three types. A fourth type of influenza, which affects only animals, also exists:

Influenza Virus A: Flus with names like H1N1 (that is, an H followed by a number, an N followed by a number) are Influenza A viruses. These are human influenza viruses of worse severity than the other types, and they are the most contagious. A-Type influenzas are the ones that undergo "antigenic shifts," mutating their genetic structures to transmit from animals to humans. These shifts also reduce human ability to produce antibodies that will fight the infections. **Pandemics are caused by A-Type influenzas.**

Influenza Virus B: Next, in decreasing severity and transmissibility, is Influenza B. B-Type influenzas mutate far more slowly than A-Types, allowing for immunities to develop among the population that prevent widespread infection.

Influenza Virus C: And as expected, Influenza C has a low level of severity and transmissibility. Type-C influenza and Type-D (below) do not mutate.

Influenza D: D-type flu viruses are a fairly recent discovery; these are influenzas isolated in animals (pigs, cattle). These are animal influenzas that do not make the jump from animal to human contagion. Of course it is theorized that mutating across species is possible, but it has not occurred and does not seem to be a factor of concern in the same way that A-Type viruses are.

Leading Up to the Spanish Flu: The Russian Flu Epidemic of 1889

Considered to be the first modern flu pandemic, the Russian Flu originated in Siberia and Kazakhstan. What allowed this influenza the dubious honor of being "first?" Again, we see that the development of civilization goes hand in hand with the spread of disease. because for the first time, transportation was sophisticated enough to permit a disease to cross vast countries and oceans. By 1889, Russia was well-equipped with a railroad system that permitted the flu to travel throughout the nation. It was during the Russian Flu's rapid spread that medical experts noticed the flu followed roads, railways and rivers, allowing them to understand that the flu was carried and spread by the movement of people, and not by more nebulous causes such as "the wind." It was an indication of things to come in the next century and an obvious but difficult lesson to learn: ease of travel doesn't apply solely to vacationers. Viruses are more than happy to take advantage of a quick trip into town.

Once the Russian Flu had reached the city of St. Petersburg, its path was clear to extend into the rest of the world. From there the flu spread to Finland and Poland, and then proceeded to infect the remainder of Europe. In a year's time the Russian Flu traveled to Africa and North America.

The death toll is estimated from 360,000 to a million people by its end. (Note: this general disagreement on the number of deaths caused by a pandemic can be seen in the calculations of the Spanish Flu's mortality. In cases of pandemic, deriving a precise number of deaths seems nearly impossible, due to factors such as misrepresentations of total numbers from countries wishing to hide their vulnerability, uncertainty as to which deaths were directly caused by the flu, and simple, general chaos in the wake of widespread illness.)

In addition to being the first modern pandemic, the Russian Flu was also the last pandemic of the 19th Century. Researchers believe it was caused by either the H3N8 or H2N2 Influenza virus. Aside from the obvious connections of both being Influenza Virus Type A, the Russian Flu pandemic relates to the Spanish Flu pandemic through an interesting speculation.

Though influenza is ordinarily a particular danger to the elderly, the Spanish Flu did not seem to behave that way, and the elderly were not *especially* at risk. It has been suggested that the older population, having already been exposed to the Russian Flu virus in 1889-1890 and its subsequent appearances through the decades that followed, may have developed some effective antibodies against the Spanish Flu.

The Spanish Flu

Where did it come from?

Like trying to pinpoint the number of fatalities in a flu pandemic, attempts to define the point of flu's origin are also subject to conjecture and argument. With the intervening factor of World War I, which had already disrupted so many of normal life's patterns, backtracking to the ground zero of the Spanish Flu pandemic becomes incredibly difficult. In hindsight, and with the ability to follow a timeline of events, combined with the knowledge we currently have developed about the way a new, deadly flu can erupt from antigenic shift, we are better able to follow a disease to its likely origins. There are three major suspects for the flu's origin:

China

For some time, the country of China was considered a likely source for the virus, because of the movement of Chinese laborers to the European battlefront, where eventually the Spanish Flu would mutate into its most deadly form. These theories have been disputed or at least diminished in importance by other arguments, however. For example, Chinese travelers entering other parts of the world did not result in any increased incidence of the flu in those areas.

Available evidence suggests that China had a relatively ordinary flu season in 1918, but this was not a convincing argument against Chinese origin. This could have been the result of one or several different elements, including:

1. that the virus began in China but had not yet mutated to its deadlier form;
2. that the virus was common enough in China that the population there had immunity; or
3. that the virus simply didn't have the legs to move through the country. At that time in China, transportation was not as sophisticated as it was in countries like the United States and Russia. As we

have discussed, this factor could have been beneficial in slowing the spread of the flu inside China.

To say definitively that the virus originated in China remains very difficult, simply because record-keeping of the time from China was highly unreliable. While reports suggest that the Chinese population faired far better than the rest of the world when it came to mortality from the Spanish Flu, these records do not extend to the smaller towns and less-populated regions where the results of the flu went unnoticed, and unrecorded.

There is also anecdotal evidence suggesting the Chinese were better able to treat flu and its complications because of their methods of treatment, including herbal and holistic treatments, which had improved throughout the centuries in response to devastating flu epidemics that had ravaged China in ancient times.

The United Kingdom, care of France

A second theory is that the Spanish Flu originated in the town of Etaples in France, where the United Kingdom had developed a hospital camp as well as a troop staging area. A new, deadly illness was found present there in 1917 (and possibly showed itself much earlier than in the camp, but was once again mistaken for another disease). This mysterious ailment was later identified as the Spanish Flu.

The incredibly crowded and busy camp was the perfect site for the spread of the contagious virus. Soldiers passed through the area at the rate of approximately 100,000 per day. The area was swampy and the camp supported a number of animals, including pigs, a common enough culprit in flu viruses transmitted from animals to humans.

Even if the flu did not originate in the United Kingdom's camp, such places were instrumental in the widespread pandemic. Countries in the midst of war were not willing to stop supplying troops to the war machine; sending sick soldiers to the front lines was preferred to quarantining them.

The United States, and the Men of Haskell County, Kansas

By far the most well-documented origin story for the Spanish Flu springs from Haskell County, Kansas. From this quiet farm community, the virus can be tracked with detective-like precision to its breeding grounds of the World War I trenches, at which point it mutated into its deadliest form. Is this merely because record-keeping was better, or because this research is easily available now? In either case, tracking the virus's progression from Haskell to the trenches of Europe is a fascinating and frightening journey.

In Haskell County, Kansas, the flu season of 1917-1918 was notably vicious. This rural farming community was stricken with a potent flu, very likely transmitted (by an antigenic shift) from sick pigs, an influenza we commonly know as "swine flu." Despite the transmissibility and morbidity of the disease, which was reported to health authorities by the local doctor, the threat of an epidemic was downplayed because of Haskell's relative remoteness. It did not seem likely that the flu would travel beyond the county and, in fact, it had seemed to pass by February 1918.

Through volunteerism and the draft, however, several young men left Haskell County to fight for the United States in World War I. They were sent first to Fort Funston, Kansas. Fort Funston was a supplementary encampment about five miles from the United States Army's base of Fort Riley, Kansas. Fort Funston was put in place to accommodate the huge numbers of new troops being brought in for training prior to their deployment overseas.

The winter of 1918 was bitterly cold. The flat plains of Kansas offer no shielding from icy winds. Against regulations, but probably out of a sense of kindness, more than 50,000 young soldiers were permitted to crowd into the heated barracks together rather than be encamped in unheated tents, exposed to the elements outdoors. It was most certainly warmer inside the barracks, but herein a few young men from Haskell County were able to share more than stories of their hometown as they gathered around the stoves with other soldiers.

The Haskell recruits arrived in Fort Funston on February 28, 1918. On the morning of March 11, a company cook, Private Albert Gitchell, reported to sick-call with flu-like symptoms; within a week, there were 500 reported infections, and within five weeks, over a thousand soldiers were sick, overwhelming the base's resources. Reports vary on the mortality of this flu outbreak, from 38 to 50 dead soldiers. At about the same time, in other parts of the United States, more flu outbreaks occurred, such as at the Ford Motor plant, and at San Quentin prison.

But again, as had been the case in Haskell, the flu seemed to recede as quickly as it had descended, and the Army's concerns were focused more on a contemporaneous measles outbreak than on the influenza. For all its severity, the influenza at the camp could have been assumed to be a bad seasonal virus worsened by close quarters and large numbers of troops.

Men from Fort Funston were transported to port cities and then put on ships to Brest, France, the incoming European port for all United States troops of the American

Expeditionary Forces. 84,000 American soldiers were sent to Europe in March 1918, and then in the following month, more than 100,000 were sent. From this point, any virus lying dormant in the body of a soldier was free to spread across the European continent in some of the most opportune environments a hungry virus could desire.

The Infection of Europe: Spring 1918

World War I is inexorably linked with Spanish Flu; as if the two world disasters came hand in hand with one another. Once American troops arrived in Brest, the dormant flu reawakened and spread to the British and French troops. On the battleground, the virus crossed the lines of no-man's land to infect the Germans and Italians. It is believed that from Italy, the virus moved into Spain.

The flu ravaged the people of Spain, including, allegedly, their king, Alfonso XIII. Obviously the flu did not originate in Spain but was dubbed the "Spanish Flu" because, thanks to their country's neutrality in the Great War, Spanish journalism was able to report uncensored accounts of the illness. News reports of the flu were first seen from Madrid in May 1918. Other countries, in the thick of the conflict, held back information on the flu in order to maintain morale among troops and civilians, and to keep enemies from spotting a weakness. This censorship served to make Spain seem like the hotbed of the illness and resulted in the pandemic being nicknamed for that country. Ironically, in Spain, the illness was called the "French Flu."

Regardless of the virus's ground zero, it is doubtless that the war played a major role in the spread and lethality of the flu. Soldiers were exhausted, underfed, and subject to tremendous strain, severely weakening their immune systems. Troops were kept in close quarters with each other and yet constantly on the move, a situation that leads to spread of disease on two levels: among units and then across the landscape, respectively. Trains full of soldiers stopped in towns along the way to their destination, soldiers disembarked and mingled, smoking, talking, and leaving the virus behind. The civilian population in Europe was also suffering its own deprivations and stresses, including the constant threat of bombing and invasion, their perilous proximity to fighting, poverty, malnutrition and outright starvation, and poor hygiene.

Movement of the flu was promoted by the vast movement of troops around the world, living in the rough conditions of trench warfare, which is a breeding ground for disease. Basically, battlegrounds consisted of a series of trenches on either side of a strip of ground known as "no-man's land." From the trenches, soldiers volleyed fire back and forth with their enemies, and were often left to wait for great stretches of anxiety-laden time, until they were able to launch from their trench in order to gain a few feet of ground further into the battlefield, ducking into another trench before being shot down.

In these unthinkable circumstances men lived, breathed, ate and slept within a few feet of each other for weeks at a time. Sanitation was impossible. Latrines were mere feet from living spaces. Mud was thick and it never dried out. Men's feet would rot in their boots. When it rained, water would stream through the trenches polluted with human waste, and in some cases, with parts of bodies that had to be abandoned in no-man's land.

And those were the conditions *without* the added trauma of flu. The virus itself so affected the activities of the troops that it was the deciding factor in battles, as in, when soldiers trapped in trench warfare might be too sick to fight, or when supplies meant for front-line fighting had to be diverted to care for the sick or dispose of the dead. It is estimated that during September through November 1918, twenty to forty percent of the U.S. Army/Navy personnel were sick with influenza or pneumonia; the flu killed more United States soldiers than the war itself.

An additional, unforeseen consequence resulted from the practices in treatment of sick soldiers. Soldiers with "mild" symptoms remained with their troops; soldiers displaying "serious" symptoms were transported to treatment centers with little or no precautions taken to quarantine them, permitting the spread of the deadlier form of the flu on a massive scale.

Soldiers sent home took the virus with them and the spread worsened.

From an infected Europe, the Spanish Flu easily moved to Africa, China, India and Russia. This was still the Spanish Flu's first wave, though, relatively mild compared to the disaster that was on the horizon, and actually by July's end, the virus seemed to be coming to the end of its run.

The Second Wave and the Deadliest Year of the Century

The Mutation

Sometime during the summer of 1918, the Spanish Flu mutated. The Second Wave tore through the warfront in Europe but also was sent around the world with thousands of soldiers returning to their homes.

Originally the "First Wave" influenza symptoms were fever, chills, nausea, aches, and diarrhea. Some victims died of secondary infections like pneumonia.

The "Second Wave" mutation brought on a whole new horror show. Symptoms were confusing and unpredictable, leading health professionals to misdiagnose the illness. Patients could present with high fevers with hallucinations, agonizing muscle pain, blindness, deafness, paralysis, vertigo, brutally fast-moving ear infections, and severe mucus membrane inflammation. Patients suffered hemorrhagic fevers, and bled from their eyes, ears, mouths and noses. Sometimes a patient could cough hard enough to tear abdominal muscles. They drowned as their lungs filled with fluids. Autopsies showed lungs that resembled the lungs of soldiers killed by poisonous gas on the battlefield.

Bizarre new symptoms arose: small pockets of air escaped from torn lung tissue and filled patients' bodies, so that when they would move, the air pockets would crackle. Some patients became so oxygen-deprived that their faces turned blue or black, resulting in the disease being nicknamed "the Blue death." When a patient turned blue, caregivers knew death was only a few hours away. The speed of the illness was like nothing that had been seen before: 48 hours from exposure to serious sickness was bad enough, but victims could sometimes die within 12 hours of first exhibiting symptoms. The symptoms were so strange and different than in many cases, medical specialists even denied that it could be the flu.

By August 1918 the virus returned to the United States in its mutated form. A ship of 200 sick people (with 4 already dead) arrived in New York City. There, the sick were taken to hospitals, but not quarantined. Similar ships fetched up in other deep port cities like Boston and New Orleans, and in foreign ports like Brest, France and Freetown, Sierra Leone, with disastrous but, in hindsight, predictable results.

Camp Devens in Massachusetts experienced a violent outbreak of the flu, and though the troop movement was restricted, officers still left the camp and went to Camp Grant in Illinois, and from Camp Grant the disease traveled to Camp Hancock in Georgia, and so on, and so on. The infirmaries of the camps were unable to handle the numbers of sick people. After receiving word that their young men were deathly ill, wives and families of sick soldiers came to visit. No precautions were taken. Visitors were taken through the forts, escorted by other sick soldiers, and were allowed to see their dying loved ones. Upon returning home, these grieving people took the Spanish Flu with them, by way of trains that traveled across the United States. Towns of every size were quickly overtaken.

Few areas of the country, or even the world, were spared from the catastrophe. If a place was accessible to outside human contact, the virus could get there as well.

The Second Wave in the United States

The Spanish Flu killed approximately 675,000 people in the United States, which is a higher death toll than the combined approximate death tolls of World War I, World War II, the Korean and Vietnamese Wars, Iraq and

Afghanistan. The majority of the deaths and the most terrifying environment created by the Spanish Flu occurred during the deadly Second Wave, from September through November 1918, with October 1918 being the deadliest month in the country's history.

Hospitals were unable to accommodate the influx of patients, and all manner of buildings (such as schools, and even private homes) were hastily converted into treatment centers. Medical professionals in 1918 did not know what caused the flu, nor did they know how to treat it or have the means to do so, beyond trying to relieve the myriad symptoms as best they could. After all, the first flu vaccine would not be available in America until the 1940s, over twenty years in the future. Not even antibiotics were developed. Penicillin's discovery was ten years away. Mechanical ventilation was not yet invented. There were no countermeasures against the flu beyond simple supportive care.

Carry a Potato in Your Pocket

Of course the public was terrified. Without any definitive answers coming from health officials regarding a cure, old wives' tales and superstitions took over, rumors of effective protection spreading and resulting in some unusual behaviors among the frightened population. Some of the measures believed to work for flu prevention and/or treatment were:

1. Bags of camphor worn around the neck (or Vicks Vapo-Rub, if it was available)
2. Gargling salt water (or Listerine)
3. Eating oranges
4. Eating sulfur
5. Putting sulfur in one's shoes
6. Burning sulfur (as a way to purify the air)
7. Teas made from things such as cedar, cherry bark, sassafras roots, elm, or pokeweed plants
8. Moonshine, or whiskey, sometimes mixed with sugar and honey
9. Doses of castor oil
10. Belladonna (sometimes used to treat colic and asthma)
11. Eating raw onions
12. Eating goosegrass
13. Keeping a potato in one's pocket.

Densely populated cities were hit the hardest, obviously, as viral infections thrive on density as a means of transmission. The United States had no treatment plan in place and the flu moved with such savage speed that it fell to local officials to attempt to protect the citizens. The ongoing war continued to be a factor in the ability to respond wisely to the pandemic. The media downplayed the seriousness of the situation, and there was general pressure to act patriotically, which certainly didn't lend itself to ordering quarantines. Any hesitation on the part of officials to act was deadly. The ferocity of the mutated virus was such that a city could be brought to its knees within 72 hours while officials were still debating what methods to employ.

Medical Mysteries During the Spanish Flu

The deadly Spanish influenza was a mystery in and of itself, and one that would not be understood until decades after it slipped into inactivity. But here, we'll look at a couple of other odd outcomes during the pandemic that remain puzzling to researchers.

The Unexpected Affliction of Young Adults and the Cytokine Storm

In 1918, America's average life expectancy dropped by twelve years.

Ordinarily, young adults are the most resistant to influenza. Strains of the flu are always known for their danger to the health-compromised, the very young or the very old. Not this time, however. No age group was safe but the uncharacteristic number of young adults (aged 20 to 35) killed by the Spanish Flu has resulted in yet another debated mystery about the disease. Unlike common physical responses to a virus, in the case of this flu, a phenomenon called a "cytokine storm" is believed to actually have killed those with strong immune systems *more easily* affected than those with weak immune systems. Ironically, then, a young, strong person was actually at a disadvantage when it came to surviving the flu.

Cytokines are an integral part of the immune system. They are regulators of the immune response, signaling to the body which cells need to activate in order to fight foreign bodies. A **cytokine storm,** then, is an overreaction by the human body in its response to the invading particles.

The immune process at work is a cycle of balance between white blood cells and the agents they release in order to fight infection. Under ordinary circumstances, inflammatory cytokines are released by white blood cells in response to an infection by a foreign body. These new cytokines, in turn, activate more white cells, until large numbers of white blood cells are activated to release inflammatory cytokines to fight the infection, which activate yet more white blood cells, which release more cytokines.

Where does it end? Well, in a balanced system, cytokines are self-regulating, containing subsets of types that "police" each other and keep matters under control. If the body is unable to regulate this system, however, autoimmune dysfunctions like cytokine storm syndrome can occur. The results can be deadly, for example, causing shock, organ failure, and systemic hyper-inflammation. Cytokine storms can be responsible for rejection of transplanted organs, and other autoimmune diseases are linked to the inability of cytokines to self-regulate. Cytokine storms often complicate respiratory diseases.

Still, the question remains as to why this influenza strain was able to goad the bodies of these young people basically into turning on themselves.

The Theory of Aspirin Poisoning

Occasionally in the research regarding the Spanish Flu, one will find "aspirin poisoning" as a subheading. Like almost every other aspect of the pandemic, this is a subject for debate.

The theory is that aspirin overdose played a role in the high death toll of the Spanish Flu. Disagreements arise pertaining to how widespread the overuse of aspirin actually was, as once more, the inconsistency of recordkeeping comes into play. Also, in comparing the death rates of populations that had access to aspirin versus those that did not, there is not enough difference in the rates that researchers can agree about the significance.

In any case, aspirin toxicity in its relationship to the Spanish Flu refers to the tendency for doctors fighting the flu to overprescribe aspirin to alleviate flu symptoms of pain and fever. There are two possible culprits associated with aspirin-relating deaths, although they are not mutually exclusive:

1. Aspirin had been trademarked in 1899 by the Bayer Company. Their patent expired in 1917, so by the time the Spanish Flu was raging across America, there were new companies producing aspirin. There was no guarantee that these companies were producing aspirin at Bayer's standards; the use of substandard or substituted ingredients may have resulted in a more dangerous product.

2. Aspirin is toxic in doses higher than four grams per day, yet doctors of 1918 prescribed doses up to 30 grams per day. The symptoms of aspirin toxicity are very much like the symptoms of the Spanish Flu, and in particular it can cause edema in the lungs, a condition that was already killing victims of the flu. Aspirin toxicity could therefore have killed outright, or worsened the deadliest symptom and hastened the death of victims.

Countermeasures

Certainly, attempts were made to slow or block the spread of the flu. Quarantines were imposed in some communities:

public places were closed (even libraries stopped lending books) and citizens were ordered to wear masks, stay indoors, and avoid physical contact with others. Public bans on spitting were issued and enforced by the police and, in New York, by Boy Scouts handing out warning cards. It begs the question of why these children were out in public at all, but the inconsistency of preventative measures was widespread.

Beyond the use of Boy Scouts, the New York City Commissioner of Health devised a plan to stagger business shifts through the city, which was meant to avoid subway overcrowding. But half-measures were no match for the mutated flu strain. In New York City, 33,000 people died before the record keepers simply stopped counting. Entire families could die within hours of one another. Morgues could not accommodate the numbers of dead, funeral parlors were overwhelmed and unable to handle the load, and cities were forced to dig mass graves to keep bodies from rotting in stacks in the streets, outside morgues, even inside homes, where the families themselves were too sick to attend to their dead.

Businesses suffered as well, forced to close because of outright quarantine or, if not, then for lack of healthy customers and workers. Vital services such as mail delivery and garbage collection were hindered or altogether ceased for a time. That winter in New England, coal deliveries were so disrupted that people froze in their own homes.

There were instances in which planning and care did work in our favor. Some cities were impressively effective in their measures. St. Louis, Missouri, for example, acted swiftly in closing schools and theaters, and banning public gatherings. As a result, the mortality rate there was significantly lower than that of hard-hit cities where quarantining had not been immediate. Portland, Oregon, set out strict curfew and quarantine rules that left them with the sad task of sending their excess coffins to other locations where they were needed.

San Francisco largely escaped the trauma of the Second Wave because of the aggressive response of the local government. All naval stations were quarantined, and they too closed all public gathering places, as had St. Louis. Citizens caught in public without masks could receive a hefty fine and be charged with disturbing the peace. This kept morbidity in the city to a minimum. The only mistake San Francisco made was assuming the flu had bypassed them, thus lifting their restrictions too early. They were infected in the Third Wave. By this time, however, the virus had again mutated and was less deadly. San Francisco's outcome was proof that response matters; when public health officials act quickly, the transmission of a disease can be brought under control, and therefore mortality significantly decreased.

Philadelphia: The Pandemic's Most Devastating Example

Philadelphia suffered the ferocity of the Second Wave more intensely than any other city in the United States and serves as a grim example of the horrors of a pandemic on an unprepared and unprotected population. Originally, Philadelphia was infected in large part by the arrival of ill sailors in the Philadelphia Navy Yard, early in the month of September 1918. The statistics alone are startling: out of Philadelphia's population of two million, at least one fourth (or, 500,000 people) contracted the flu; there were 16,000 flu-related deaths overall with 12,000 of those occurring in September, October and November 1918. Let's examine the reasons why Philadelphia in particular was hit so hard.

The first two reasons were, to different extents, war-related:

1. A large percentage of qualified medical personnel were serving the war effort. It is estimated that 25% of Philadelphia's doctors, and an even higher percentage of its nurses, were stationed overseas, as well as were hundreds of trained medical workers. Therefore, when the flu spread outside of military installations,

the civilian medical establishment was markedly understaffed.

2. Demand for supplies and industry for the war effort (i.e., the steel industry, for which Philadelphia was already known, and shipbuilding and munitions) dramatically increased labor demand. At this promise of opportunity, a flood of workers arrived in the city including two vastly underprivileged populations: African Americans wishing to escape the dangers of the southern United States; and European immigrants fleeing their war-torn countries. This led to a crisis in housing, as thousands of people crowded into filthy, cramped tenement districts. (It is, in effect, the same overcrowding and sanitation issues that caused the uprising of workers after the Industrial Revolution -- but this level of rebellion had not yet come to Philadelphia.) By 1918 Philadelphia's steel mills employed thousands, which turned into massive overcrowding in impoverished slums, where people shared outhouses, beds, apartments, filthy water and terrible air quality. Like the trenches on the European battlefields, thickly crowded tenement housing is in and of itself a health crisis, and a situation ripe for the spread of infection.

We can clearly see that Philadelphia was an open invitation for severe influenza infection. The third reason for Philadelphia's devastation was now in the hands of the authorities. The path for the pandemic was left wide open by the city's health officials, who failed to recognize or act upon the danger that was at their doorstep.

600 soldiers were ill at the Philadelphia Navy Yard, and among the civilians, the first cases of infection were reported. Yet once again, the war effort took precedence in the minds of officials, and we know this is not the first or last time that this bad bargain was made during the Spanish Flu Pandemic, as the trenches in Europe themselves were fed with thousands of sick soldiers.

The Fourth Liberty Loan Campaign was set to occur on September 28, 1918. Despite knowing that crowds and public events should be avoided, the Department of Public Health and Charities gave little or no resistance to the idea of going forward with the event, going so far as to attribute the fatalities to that point as a result of seasonal flu rather than to the deadly pandemic. The Fourth Liberty Loan Campaign would go forward as planned. This rousing, patriotic celebration was meant to inspire the public to purchase war bonds and included a parade and a concert in Philadelphia's Willow Grove Park. Some 200,000 Philadelphians gathered in the streets for the festivities. The campaign was obviously a great success as well over \$500 million dollars in war bonds were purchased.

Within three days of the campaign, over 600 new cases of the flu were reported among civilians, and this was only the beginning: 2,600 cases were reported during the second week of October; twice that many the week after. Schools, saloons, theaters and public gatherings were finally closed, but far too late to curb the damage that had already been done.

Among the population, flu contagion affected race and gender equally; no particular group seemed less vulnerable to catching the virus. Death rates, however, were much higher in the poorer communities, for the obvious reasons that proper care was simply less available to them. In the terror of the time, immigrants were scapegoated for the spread of the disease, singled out as having poor hygiene or morals.

Hospitals were overwhelmed by the sheer numbers of patients, which far exceeded the expected capacity. Philadelphia General Hospital, for example, had the capacity for 2,000 patients but was coping with 3,400 by mid-October. Volunteers were desperately needed and difficult to find. Public terror of the disease made most people unwilling to assist even in a neighborly capacity. Because the flu killed so many young adults, children were frequently orphaned, and even if they were not sick themselves, were left to starve because others dared not approach them for fear of contagion.

But some volunteer help was found. Doctors and nurses came out of retirement to assist. Religious and civic organizations were the main source of voluntary help. Medical and nursing schools closed and the students were sent forward as if they were fully trained, to work as best they could in the chaotic circumstances. In a faint silver lining, social barriers were broken down by the sheer need of the city. Women who were accustomed to an upper class lifestyle could find themselves walking through blood in a hospital ward as they tried to change bedsheets, and worked side by side with working-class citizens. Prominent Philadelphian women, rising to solve problems that their government could not seem to fix, united together to seek aid for their city, and together set up soup kitchens and food delivery.

The city's infrastructure was utterly unequipped to handle the number of corpses. There were not even enough coffins for the number of corpses -- and terrified gravediggers refused to work. While morgues were filled with stacks of bodies and emergency morgues were established, the circumstances were so desperate that corpses were often left to rot for days, not only in the streets, but within the very tenements where the victims had lived. People were often too ill themselves to dispose of, or even move, the bodies of the dead. Families might have to live in the same apartment as a dead body for days at a time.

After a nightmarish three months, the Spanish Flu seemed to recede from Philadelphia of its own volition. Incidences of infection and death began to decrease sharply after November, leaving behind a shocked city to pick up the pieces.

The Long Ending

Armistice and the Third Wave

On November 11, 1918, an Armistice was signed to bring World War I fighting to an end, and coincidentally, this seemed to coincide with the lessening of the deadly Second Wave of flu. Unfortunately the celebration of Armistice Day resulted in huge gatherings of crowds for parties and parades. Thousands of soldiers were returning to their homes. This sudden increase in socialization and travel caused the Third Wave of flu to sweep through the United States and the rest of the world. Even President Woodrow Wilson is believed to have contracted the flu during negotiations for the Treaty of Versailles, to end the war, in the early months of 1919.

Research and details on the Third Wave of the Spanish Flu serve as a sort of active example of the attitude toward the flu at the time. The Third Wave is the least documented phase of the Spanish Flu, as if the world at large was simply too exhausted by the Second Wave to pay it much attention. Even now, in the writings and films consulted to write this overview, the Third Wave is simply an addendum, summarized quickly, and saying, basically, "The Third Wave was worse than the First Wave but not nearly as bad as the Second Wave."

Indeed, and thankfully, the virus had mutated once more into something less deadly. Sparing its victims the outright terror of the Second Wave, the Third Wave seems to recede in memory, giving way to the celebration of the end of World War I. Ironically, the celebration of the war's end was a major factor in the Third Wave's eruption. Perhaps in people's minds, the end of the war equaled the end of the flu, as if Armistice also meant that the virus could no longer spread.

In the United States, the Third Wave had the greatest effect on the western and southwestern United States. Outside the United States, the world also suffered the Third Wave, which despite bringing its own share of deaths, simply did not receive the attention of the Second Wave. The attention span for this tragedy had ended and the world was ready to move on from a terrible time in history. As we have learned, however, influenza viruses operate on their own timeline, regardless of the amount of attention humans choose to give them.

The Third Wave hovered over the world for about another year; there are reports of cases and deaths happening as late as 1920.

Medical Advances Made During the Spanish Flu Pandemic

When discussing what medical advances were made as a result of the Spanish Flu pandemic, a phrase that comes to mind is "Better late than never." This may be true, as the really significant advances happened after -- sometimes decades after -- the pandemic, yet it also implies that doctors and researchers during the pandemic did little to help. But what, actually, could they have done?

To the medical community, the Spanish Flu was an impossible opponent during its reign of terror. The flu came on too fast and too hard to be concurrently studied, the science was not available for understanding or research, and anyone who came within an arm's reach of the illness was at risk of catching it. Even the common-sense lessons regarding contagion and safety seem to have been learned (or at least, applied) only after it was too late, in many cases. Quarantining, the most obvious preventative measure, was ignored in favor of the war effort.

No significant medical advances were made during the waves of the pandemic, except possibly one rudimentary discovery. By the pandemic's end, it had been ascertained that a blood transfusion from a survivor was an effective treatment method. We can understand now that this was because through their blood, a survivor could transfer antibodies for the virus into the body of the victim, or in loose terms, this was a very early and inconvenient type of vaccination. Vaccinations were understood, at least. A smallpox vaccination had been in use for decades.

The problems that kept this transfusion treatment from being useful on a large scale were those of logistics and safety. Blood transfusion was still accomplished only directly by donor-to-patient interaction. Survivors would have to be present and physically hooked up to the suffering victim in order for this procedure to even begin. Blood typing, too, was only understood at a basic level, thus the risks of the procedure might outweigh the benefits, should the wrong blood factors be matched.

What could not be accomplished in medical advancement during the Spanish Flu was done in the years that followed. Perhaps the world wanted to leave the Spanish Flu in the past, but scientists wanted a better understanding of the pandemic, if only to know how to prevent its happening again.

A Silver Lining: Women's Increased Status in the Fallout of Flu and War

We have already seen how thoroughly the flu ravaged the soldiers sent to, and returning from, fighting in the war. In the desperate plight of Philadelphia, we have learned how many women stepped forward in the crisis to care for their city when it seemed no one else could. The combination of these trends -- the death of men, the actions of women -- added unforeseen momentum toward achieving women's rights in the United States. The suffragette movement had begun in 1913, and reached its crescendo with the end of the war, at which time women were more than proving their right to a place in the country's democracy.

It is little surprise that the flu killed a disproportionate number of men, because it spread through the world on the backs of soldiers. In the United States in 1918, 175,000 more men died than women. That number, in connection with the fatalities and absences caused by war, created a labor shortage in the United States. Women stepped in to fill the gaps, working outside their homes in numbers never before seen. After the war, the number of women in the workplace was 25% higher than it had been before. They were found capable of working in the roles previously held only by men (especially manufacturing and textile industry jobs), and proved themselves even further in a period already ripe for societal change, including the women's suffrage movement.

Being a part of the workforce allowed women to gain independence, both social and financial, that had been previously unknown. Women took positions of leadership in military, police forces and in industry. Women were able to command respect and make decisions in their lives that we now take quite for granted. Civil organizations sprang up to support the cause. For example, the National Federation of Business and Professional Women's Clubs was founded in 1919. The goals of this organization were equal pay, equal rights, and an end to sex discrimination in employment.

Politicians were forced to take note of women's increased decision-making power. President Woodrow Wilson declared women to be "partners" of not only the war effort but the economy itself, and he declared that they should be afforded the right to vote. The 19th Amendment would be ratified two years later (in August 1920). By 1925, Wyoming had elected Nellie Taylor Ross as the United States' first female governor.

Stories
from the Spanish Flu

In 2008, in commemoration of the 90th anniversary of the Spanish Flu Pandemic, the CDC invited members of the public to send them their recollections of the time. From those they put together a "storybook" of accounts from the time of the flu. This is available at CDC.gov and contains poignant, frightening and sometimes even humorous tales from those who were impacted by the pandemic. Contributors who were actually alive during the pandemic were over 90 years old when the website's materials were gathered. Many other contributors were children or grandchildren of those who lived, or died, during the pandemic, sharing the stories that were handed down to them, and in a sad number of these anecdotes, the storytellers were orphaned by the pandemic, and they tell tales of parents they never knew.

Though each story is individual to its teller, they share many striking similarities. Storytellers recall:

1. Rumors of illness in Europe, stories of soldiers dead in such numbers that their bodies were burned rather than buried, or of a spreading sickness in large nearby cities. Yet little information came in the form of concrete evidence or advice. Word of the pandemic seemed to spread more slowly than the pandemic itself, or on pace with it, as it arrived on the same trains that brought the bad news.

2. More than one storyteller recalls the horrifying speed of the illness; that people could die so quickly made the situation feel unreal. The shock of losing so many people so fast was often more incapacitating than grief itself. Bodies had to be buried so quickly that there was no time to adjust to the loss.

3. Large families were ill together, lucky if at least one of them (sometimes a child) was well enough to care for the rest. Some families died together, admitted one by one to emergency care stations over the course of a week or two, or alone in their

home, unable to get help or attend each other. There are tales of mothers losing four children in a month. Survival seemed like a matter of luck; clearly the storytellers themselves made it through but they talk of lost parents, siblings, and friends, and to this day wonder what those lives would have been like, if not cut short by the pandemic.

4. Those who actually suffered but survived the pandemic describe the severity of the sickness, saying that they were never again as sick in their lives as they were when they had Spanish Flu.

5. Families experienced terrible economic hardship, particularly when the breadwinner (usually the father) died. Children were sent away to live with relatives and often separated from their own siblings. Families often had to be split apart, sometimes losing contact with each other for years or even the rest of their lives, as name changes and the fleeing public put too much distance between parted young siblings for them ever to find each other again. Other families lived with guilt after sending the children of relations away to orphanages, when they were simply unable to take on the burden or three or four more children in their own home.

6. Those storytellers who were hardly more than infants at the time of the pandemic can recall grim imagery that affected them for the rest of their lives: the sounds and sights of hearses passing by their homes, full hospitals and emergency aid stations set up by the Red Cross; coffins arriving by the trainload, burials delayed because gravediggers were unable or unwilling to keep up with demand, deathly ill parents in bed for days at a time, or alternatively, relatives who were well one day and dead 48 hours later, and the awful sight of dead bodies lying on the streets. They remember community churches unable to keep up with the sheer number of funerals, and schools used to house corpses. One gravedigger recalled spending an entire day digging graves for one family of six. One woman recalls her mother, a seamstress, staying up all night to sew shrouds for the dead.

7. Communities that would, under ordinary circumstances, care for their members in need, were unable to do so as resources were insufficient to meet the unexpected demands.

Some of the stories are more specific.

1. Many soldiers recount their experiences at infected camps. One was given the duty of "dosing" dying

soldiers with whiskey. Another was put on burial duty when he himself was sick with the flu; he recalls there were 700 dead that needed to be buried.

2. Memories are shared of a mother who voluntarily helped care for flu victims, risking (and sadly, sacrificing) her own life in taking care of others.

3. One woman's grandfather, who was a seminary student, was assigned to take a horse-drawn cart through streets, calling out to collect bodies from homes. He believes seminary students were selected because there was simply no one else who could, or would, do the task. She remembers her grandfather as a small man who probably had much difficulty moving bodies. He did the work for months, but never caught the flu.

4. Another storyteller recalls the time when as a child she visited a graveyard with her mother, and asked why so many of the tombstones had the same date of death; she learned that day from her grandmother that many members of her own family had died during the pandemic.

5. A doctor from Wyoming, treating his patients with rotgut whiskey (to cough the phlegm out) actually stole evidentiary bootlegger's whiskey from the sheriff's department when his own supply ran out.

6. Another tells of a family delighted by a visit from their son who was with the Army, not realizing that he had brought the influenza home with him. Shortly after he left to return to his base, the entire family fell ill. The soldier survived, but many of his family members did not.

A touching number of these stories conclude with the storyteller's admission that these personal experiences, or the tales of their grandparents or parents, led them to work in the field of healthcare, influenza preparedness and promotion of vaccinations.

With memories this long-lasting and vivid, passed down through generations, it seems strange that the Spanish Flu is sometimes considered the "forgotten pandemic." But even within the tales told in the CDC's storybook lies this occasional admission from a survivor: we just wanted to forget.

The "Forgotten Pandemic"?

It seems impossible to believe that a worldwide tragedy of these proportions could be "forgotten," but the truth remains that the Spanish Flu faded purposefully from the public's minds and attention.

What are some reasons why the Spanish Flu was downplayed and quickly forgotten by the public, until the reemergence of the virus in the 1990s and 2000s?

1. **The flu moved and killed rapidly.** Media of the time was unable to keep up with the pace of the pandemic and in more rural areas around the world, the flu might not be reported at all, and its outcome never recorded. What's more, in light of wartime politics, news blackouts, censorship and the overall inability to keep good records hindered what potency the media might have had.

2. **Deadly illness was common.** The population was accustomed to the ravages of other pandemics that had arisen in the decades just before and after the flu outbreak, including cholera, diphtheria, yellow fever, and typhoid fever. In the local sense, another "pandemic" received no more attention than its predecessors.

3. **World War I was the major focus**. When flu news and fatalities were reported alongside news of the war's deaths and drama, the flu may have been seen as merely another facet of the war's horrors. And while the flu moved quickly and brutally, the war had been waging for four years before the onset of the flu pandemic. With the end of the war came the end of public attention to the flu, and a desire to focus on the future.

Biological Warfare: Outing the Spanish Flu

The Research that Followed

In 1918, both the study of, and the understanding of, viruses and infections was so unsophisticated it was helpless, and for many years following the pandemic, science could only point to patterns and symptoms as they were understood at the time. The virus had been lethal; its effects brutally impacted people around the world; these were results but not explanations. Many medical authorities of 1918 believed the cause of the pandemic to have been bacterial, as the existence of viruses had not yet been discovered. By and large, the Spanish Flu was blamed on "Pfeiffer's bacillus," (currently known as Haemophilus influenzae, bacteria that can cause severe infections such as pneumonia and meningitis, particularly in very young children).

The Spanish Flu remained enigmatic for decades following its pandemic, with no one able to ascertain what specifically caused its lethality, its origins, or what health officials might be able to do to defend against future pandemics.

As science caught up with the questions, researchers (and those dramatically known as "virus hunters") began to search for a way to recreate the Spanish Flu virus in order to divine its secrets. Only then could we know how, or if, we could stop calamities of its magnitude.

The hunt was subject to the passage of time and the progress of technology. It began with simple steps:

1. By 1931, Vanderbilt University figured out how to grow an influenza virus inside chicken eggs (but recall, this was not the Spanish flu virus, rather it was seasonal flu). This odd-sounding task was a medical victory because it meant influenza samples need not be obtained from the sick. The studied samples helped researchers define the differences between A-Type and B-Type flus. (Of note, growing viruses in chicken eggs is a practice that continues well into the 21st century.)

2. By 1936, two more steps toward understanding had been taken. Researcher Richard Shope had made great strides in understanding the relationship between swine flu and its transfer to humans, showing the ease with which both the flu and the antibodies to it could be shared between pigs and their keepers.

3. Meanwhile, the invention of the electron microscope permitted researchers to see what they had only been able to theorize before: that indeed, there were smaller particles than germs at work.

With the combined ability to grow viruses in the lab, to understand their differences, and to literally see their characteristics under electron microscope, researchers were able to start work on a flu vaccine. Testing had shown that immunity for flu viruses is specific, and that antibodies for one strain of the flu virus will not work on another. The solution seems simple enough: more than one type of antibody was included in the vaccine, a practice that remains in effect today. The first uses of an influenza vaccine were in 1944 (for military personnel, and just in time for the United States' entry into World War II) and 1945 (for civilians).

Ultimately, searching for methods to prevent influenza has influenced a) the development of vaccines for other illnesses, and b) other areas of research in genetic coding and chemicals.

Finding the Real Spanish Flu Virus

The Spanish Flu virus is extinct, and for this, we can consider ourselves lucky. Those who wished to study it, however, needed a genetic sample of "the real thing." When technology was ready to safely investigate the deep inner workings of this influenza, it was long gone.

The researchers had to approach the task in much the same way that dinosaurs could be brought back to life in *Jurassic Park* - without the merchandising, perhaps. The genetic material had to be located somehow and then replicated under extremely careful conditions. But where does one find the genetic material of a virus that has been gone for almost a century? Tissue samples from its victims were the only option. The question then became: where can one find tissue samples from 1918 that have not completely decomposed beyond usefulness?

Brevig Mission's Grim Treasure. *Brevig Mission in Alaska was the key to the discovery, recreation and then dismantling of the virus. This small fishing village lies on the Bering Sea, northwest of Nome, closer to Russia than it is to Anchorage. In 1918, Brevig Mission was populated by 80 adults, most of whom were Inuit natives. Debate* *remains as to how the Spanish influenza virus managed to reach this remote location, but two possibilities are clear: the town was visited by traders and the town had mail delivery.*

From November 15 through November 20, 1918, 72 of the village's 80 adults died from the Spanish Flu. The tragedy was marked by a mass grave in which all the victims were buried together. The grave had one notable, unknown benefit: in the permafrost ground of Alaska, the bodies remained frozen and did not decompose.

Johan Hultin, Microbiologist Adventurer. In 1951, microbiologist Johan Hultin (who was dashing sort of intellectual, a skier, hiker, and builder; rather like the Indiana Jones of Iowa) went to Brevig Mission in hopes of obtaining samples of the 1918 virus. He received permission from the village elders to exhume the grave and obtain tissue samples. Within the mass grave he found the bodies well intact and he was indeed able to obtain several samples of lung tissue. The problem, however, was transporting the tissue from Brevig Mission back to the University of Iowa, a journey he took by DC-3 propeller plane. At the time, there was no means to transport the frozen tissue. Hultin actually attempted to refreeze the tissue samples each time his plane stopped to refuel, by using the carbon dioxide from fire extinguishers. Eventually upon his return to Iowa, Hultin found himself unable to get the virus to grow under lab conditions. Remarkably, this was not the end of Hultin's part in outing the killer flu.

A Second Chance.   Still, it would be almost fifty years before Hultin revisited Brevig Mission. The idea for returning to the fishing village's mass gravesite came to him when he learned that Jeffery Taubenberger, a molecular pathologist for the Armed Forces Institute of Pathology, had managed to obtain a tissue sample from a 1918 victim and partially map the Spanish Flu virus's RNA in the late 1990s. In Dr. Taubenberger's case, his tissue sample had been taken from a young soldier who died from influenza and pneumonia at Fort Jackson, South Carolina in 1918.   The soldier's tissue was expressly collected and preserved for later study.   Dr. Taubenberger and his group made quite significant progress with the sample, including learning that the deadly flu was an Influenza A type. But their RNA sequencing was incomplete and many questions remained unanswered.

Johan Hultin contacted Dr. Taubenberger to offer his input: the Brevig Mission site was likely still intact and samples could be obtained there. Taubenberger's research group was interested in samples, yet Hultin, who was by then 72 years old, paid for the trip to Brevig Mission himself, and also took his own personal tools (including gardening shears) in order to perform the tissue gathering. He obtained permission once more to unearth the burial site and used local workers to help him dig. In this excavation, he discovered a corpse he nicknamed "Lucy," a young woman who died in 1918 from virus complications. The permafrost had kept her lungs completely intact and frozen perfectly. This time, Hultin was able to ship the tissue to Taubenberger's research group. In Lucy's lungs, positive genetic material from the 1918 virus was found.

Eventually, decoding the Spanish Flu's full-length gene sequence would be accomplished with three tissue samples: that of Lucy, that of the Fort Jackson soldier and that of a service member who died from acute respiratory failure as a result of the virus in September 1918. Researchers of the Armed Forces Institute of Pathology decoded the gene sequence.

Why is the genetic sequencing important?

Through genetic sequencing, scientists were able to develop a family tree for the Spanish Flu, linking it to classic swine influenza strains, and noting too that it differed significantly from current strains of avian flu. Eventually it was theorized that this particular virus moved from birds to mammals, such as swine, and then to humans, but bird-flu tissue samples prior to 1918 simply do not exist, so that remains uncertain. Still, the virus continued to be elusive in some areas, as researchers were unable to determine what characteristics made it: a) so deadly and b) so contagious. Ordinary markers and obvious genetic features one would expect to find in highly virulent illnesses were not present in the Spanish Flu's genetic code.

Once the genome of the 1918 virus was sequenced, a live version of the virus could be constructed.

But, why would they want to do that? Wasn't it incredibly risky? Yes, but the genetic coding still left questions unanswered. Only in live virus testing could researchers observe the behaviors of the virus and single out the characteristics that made it so dangerously virulent.

The reconstruction of the live virus would require the creation of plasmids, which are elements used in genetic engineering. Plasmids are non-essential molecular material, which can function like little 3-D printers to transfer genetic material and regenerate genetic sequences. Once the Spanish Flu virus had been genetically decoded, eight plasmids were made to replicate its eight genetic strands by researchers at Mount Sinai.

Creating a Lethal Virus

You might be relieved to know that reconstruction of the deadliest flu virus in the 20th century was not undertaken carelessly. The CDC Headquarters in Atlanta was the chosen location of the reconstruction, and Biosecurity Level 3 practices were employed, as well as additional measures, to enforce the protection of everyone involved, from the workers in direct contact with the virus to the surrounding environment and the community.

In researching biologically hazardous materials, there are four "biosafety levels" that are employed, each level corresponding to the level of risk that would be posed by research. Level One Biosafety corresponds to the lowest degree of risk, and Level Four Biosafety to the highest degree of risk. For each of these risk levels there are also corresponding standards of practice and equipment, and even laboratory facilities that are situation-appropriate. For each risk level there are also primary and secondary barriers of protection. Primary barriers are specific to handling the materials (gloves, masks, special storage containers) and secondary barriers are air filtration systems and even the design of the laboratory.

Only one person was permitted to work on the actual *reconstruction* of the virus. That was Dr. Terrence Tumpey, a microbiologist who was hired by the CDC to study influenza viruses. As added precautions, Dr. Tumpey was required to work alone, after hours, when all other employees had left the labs. His work was protected by fingerprint scan and by iris scan. As he worked on the project, he took daily doses of influenza antiviral drug, but he was also made aware that if he became infected, he would be quarantined. Dr. Tumpey accepted these risks in order to perform his groundbreaking work on bringing an extinct virus back to life.

Dr. Tumpey used reverse genetics to grow cell cultures of the virus from the plasmids that had been created from the 1918 sample. These plasmids were introduced to human kidney cells, as his colleagues and the scientific world waited in July 2005, Dr. Tumpey attempted to produce the RNA of the complete virus. When at last he succeeded, researchers knew that they could now plumb the secrets of the Spanish Flu.

The Live Virus: Available for Interrogation

Study of the Spanish Flu virus was designated as a Biosecurity Level 3 and the careful restrictions that this included were as follows:

1. Personnel were required to wear double gloves, scrubs, shoe covers, surgical gowns, and an air-purifying respirator.
2. Personnel were required to shower before exiting the lab.
3. All work with the virus was performed in a biosafety cabinet (the design of which is certified).

4. Laboratory airflow was filtered and controlled to prevent airborne travel of the virus.

5. Work with the 1918 virus could not be performed alongside work with other flu viruses.

In identifying the genes of a virus that make it dangerous, along with the genes that make it vulnerable, scientists were able to target subsequent vaccines and antiviral drugs to these specific factors. Vaccination and antivirals are on the front lines of preparedness for pandemics.

What was learned from the reconstructed virus?

The reconstructed virus showed itself to be highly adept at quick replication. The reconstructed virus was 100 times more lethal in lab mice than other viruses tested. That much was probably expected. Also, it was of interest to researchers that the 1918 virus only attacked the lungs, but not other organs of the body. The grouping of genes also weakened the bronchial tubes and lungs of victims, practically an open invitation for bacterial pneumonia.

But more specifically, tests on laboratory mice showed that four days after infection, the amount of replicated cells of the Spanish Flu virus remarkably higher than that of seasonal flu viruses. This outcome was replicated by infecting human lung cells with the virus, showing that the 1918 virus could produce up to 50 times the amount of virus as comparison viruses. These results suggested that the polymerase genes in the 1918 virus were a notable part of its transmissibility. Polymerase is an enzyme responsible for replication in a genetic code. This discovery led to development and clinical trials of antiviral drugs that specifically targeted polymerases.

The "HA" gene was significantly responsible for the virus's lethality. Genetically swapping out the Spanish Flu's HA gene with that of seasonal viruses returned its behavior to that of seasonal flus. The HA gene is the hemagglutinin gene mentioned previously, which provides the "H__" aspect of naming A-Type Influenza viruses. The Spanish Flu was designated as H1N1.

Ultimately, the work of Dr. Tumpey and his colleagues would show that there was no *single* factor that made the Spanish Flu into the notoriously dangerous A-Type that it was, but a perfect storm of characteristics that, when combined, produced an unprecedented, killer flu virus. Dr. Tumpey's description called the genes of the virus a "constellation" that produced a deadly outcome.

One Hundred Years Since Then

People may have been eager to forget the 1918 pandemic, but viruses operate on their own schedule and are not subject to flagging morale. The world suffered three more influenza pandemics in the century following the Spanish Flu. Though no pandemic comes free of damage, the world was lucky that none of the three were as severe, widespread or deadly as 1918's flu. The influenza pandemics were:

1. **The Asian Flu, 1957-1958 (H2N2),** which killed more than one million people worldwide with some estimates being closer to two million, came in two waves. A vaccine was developed and made available quickly, which helped contain the pandemic. H2N2 remained in the seasonal flu circulation for ten years

until it mutated (by antigenic shift) into H3N2 in 1968, causing a new pandemic.

2. **The Hong Kong Flu, 1968-1969 (H3N2),** killed more than one million people worldwide. It is believed that the flu entered the United States through troops returning from Vietnam. The Hong Kong Flu was a less deadly virus than the Asian Flu, which might be because it evolved from the Asian Flu and some immunity was in the population at large. The presence of antibiotics helped stave of secondary infections, and medical care was more readily available to support those who were ill.

3. **The Swine Flu, 2009-2010 (H1N1).** A descendant of the Spanish Flu, this complex virus arrived showing a mixture of human, bird and two types of swine viruses. Like its deadly predecessor, the Swine Flu seems readily able to infect young adults and often results in secondary pneumonia. An interesting statistic is that the estimated number of people who contracted this virus is actually greater than the number infected by the Spanish Flu (a great increase in the world's population since 1918 can account for this), but the mortality rate of the Swine Flu does not appear to be significantly greater than that of seasonal flus. This time period was also when surprising similarities were discovered between the 2009 H1N1

virus and the 1918 H1N1 virus, and that the vaccine released in 2010-2011 (which included 2009 H1N1 virus) would work to immunize against the 1918 virus.

4. **Avian Influenza A (H7N9).** Currently the avian influenza virus (the "bird flu") is a pressing concern among scientists; it is a quite deadly Type-A influenza strain with a fatality rate of about 39%. The one thing that keeps it from becoming a pandemic is its highly limited transmissibility -- it does not move easily from human to human. Most cases of the illness have resulted from human contact with birds (poultry farmers, for example). Should it mutate into a form with increased transmissibility, experts feel it could cause a pandemic every bit as deadly as the Spanish Flu.

How Safe Are We From an Influenza Pandemic?

The answer to this question seems to be a mixed message.

We Know What to Do

Medically, we seem to be capable of fighting disease. We know the causes, the answers. We have the technology in place to dissect a virus down to its RNA. Globally, we are better equipped to fight illness than were the people of 1918.

Diagnostic testing is now available and laboratories are able to produce test results quickly. Each year, flu vaccines are updated and made available to the public. Antiviral drugs have been developed that can not only treat the flu, but can also serve as preventative measures. Antibiotics are able to treat secondary infections.

Devoted organizations spearhead the fight against pandemics. The Global Influenza Surveillance and Response System (GISRS) is a division of the World Health Organization (WHO) that monitors seasonal flus for any changes and watches for the emergence of new human influenza viruses; centers around the world collaborate with GISRS to collect specimens to track influenza outbreaks. Countries are requested to notify WHO within 24 hours of detecting any novel Influenza Type-A virus; this is essential practice for quick identification of influenza viruses with pandemic potential. The Influenza Division of the CDC evaluates influenza viruses to promote the effectiveness of annual flu vaccines. For example, when the 2009 H1N1 pandemic struck, they focused study on this strain with the goals of understanding the complete spectrum of H1N1 illnesses as well as their transmissibility. H1N1 viruses were found to have increased morbidity when compared with seasonal influenza.

But, are we willing and able to do it?

Unfortunately the world is not protected from the possibility of pandemic. The matter of population alone has put us at risk. Not only has our world's population grown to over seven billion people, but so have the numbers of swine and poultry required to feed us all. The opportunity for a novel influenza virus has grown right alongside these bulging populations. With the increased number of people who can get sick, a pandemic is bound to tax the medical system every bit as much as it did in 1918, and the CDC and WHO have issued many warnings and guidelines in dealing with this risk. Their recommendations have been followed to varying extents throughout the world.

Another disadvantage we have in the face of contagion is our incredible ease of travel. In 1918, a voyage across the Atlantic Ocean might take two weeks; we are now able to fly around in the world in a matter of hours, taking our viruses right along with us. Thanks to the ever-increasing mobility of humanity, exotic pathogens like Ebola virus have found their way out of the wilderness and directly into populated areas.

The current "best defense" against pandemic influenza is a vaccine. Vaccines have their own challenges: first, that they are not 100% effective even when they're well-matched to current virus strains; and second, it can take as long as 20 weeks to develop and manufacture a new vaccine. This is highly inconvenient timing, as a pandemic can sweep around the world in 20 weeks, as we know from the travels of the Spanish Flu.

Even with the luck of a vaccine's creation come the logistical problems of 1) making enough for everyone and 2) distributing it to those who need it. One cannot exactly ask all infected people to pop in for their shot at the CDC lab. A possible solution is a kind of medical unicorn, the "universal vaccine," something that would inoculate against all types of influenza virus Type A, but until that is discovered, researchers seek better and faster ways to produce the vaccines we do have.

Practically speaking, all the knowledge we have gathered is of little use without cooperation from governments, the media, and individuals. Excessive preparedness might seem like a waste of tax dollars right up until the moment it is desperately needed.

Conclusion: Centennial

O n May 7, 2018, the 100-year anniversary of the 1918 influenza pandemic, the CDC, along with the Rollins School of Public Health at Emory University, conducted a symposium. Experts from around the world gathered to discuss both pandemic preparedness and the current pandemic threats. Innovation comes from collaboration. An influenza virus does not pause to respect social, political or geographical lines. As with any challenge to humanity, the best hopes of victory lie in recognizing the problem, and working together, beyond the imaginary lines of borders and ideology, toward the solution.

Resources

Films

"Deadliest Plague of the 20th Century: Spanish Flu of 1918." Daily Documentary Channel.

"Kiss of the Spanish Lady." *Turning Points of History* (2001). Directed by Denise Poirier.

Books/Articles

Barry, John M. The Great Influenza: The Epic Story of the Deadliest Plague in History. New York: Viking, 2004.

Blackburn, Christine Crudo, and Gerald W. Parker and Morten Wendelbo. "How the 1918 Flu Pandemic Helped Advance Women's Rights." (2018) Smithsonianmag.com.

Byerly, Carol R. "The U.S. Military and the Influenza Pandemic of 1918-1919." www.ncbi.nlm.nih.gov.

Cheng, K.F. "What happened in China during the 1918 influenza pandemic?" International Journal of Infectious Diseases. Volume 11, Issue 4, July 2007: 360–364.

Duda, Kristina. "Why are Some Flu Seasons Worse Than Others?" (2019) verywellhealth.com.

He D, Dushoff J, Day T, Ma J, Earn DJ (September 2013). "Inferring the causes of the three waves of the 1918 influenza pandemic in England and Wales". Proceedings. Biological Sciences. 280 (1766).

Jordan, Douglas. "Ask a CDC Scientist: Dr. Terrance Tumpey and the Reconstruction of the 1918 Pandemic Virus." CDC.gov.

Jordan, Douglas. "The Deadliest Flu: The Complete Story of the Discovery and Reconstruction of the 1918 Pandemic Virus." CDC.gov.

Rosenberg, Jennifer. "1918 Spanish Flu Pandemic" 2019. Thoughtco.com.

Taubenberger JK, Morens DM (January 2006). "1918 Influenza: the mother of all pandemics". Emerging Infectious Diseases. 12 (1): 15–22.

Wallace, Rob. "Medical Innovations: From the 1918 Pandemic to a Flu Vaccine." (2020) nationalww2museum.org.

Wirth, Thomas. "Influenza: 'Spanish Flu' Pandemic, 1918-19. (2011) Philadelphiaencyclopedia.org.

Websites

"Pandemic Influenza Storybook." CDC.gov

"Pandemics that Changed History." History.com

"Spanish Flu." History.com